Cocktails and More

Cardiac Emergency

A Book on Heart Attack and Its Management

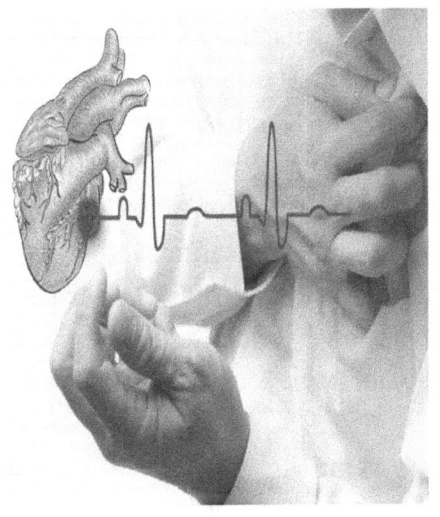

By

Paolo Jose de Luna

Les Ilagan

Cocktails and More

Table of Contents

Introduction - A Cardiac Emergency

Chest pain is nothing new since it's a common complaint made by various people. It can come from a sudden bout of fullness after a heavy meal, but it can also come from trauma or from a respiratory disease like pneumonia. But when chest pain settles in that's excruciating and unbearable, along with difficulty of breathing and an extreme case of sweating, then you know there's something wrong here.

Heart attack or *myocardial infarction*, as it is termed in the healthcare setting, is a condition wherein the heart doesn't get a sufficient amount of oxygen to support its consistent function. This is often due to the constriction of the coronary arteries, the tiny arteries that provide blood supply to the heart muscles, or a clog in the coronary arteries. When this happens, the heart doesn't get its supply of oxygen and the heart muscles can get damaged. It only takes a few minutes for the heart to survive without oxygen and in about a mere 3-5 minutes, the heart can get sustain damage called "ischemia".

The heart can only go for so long without oxygen. Oftentimes, those who sustain a prolonged heart attack or myocardial infarction are left with irreversible cardiac damage that may show as signs and symptoms like easy fatigability, abnormal heart rhythms, a faster or slower heart rate, and a radiating chest pain. With these alarming signs and symptoms, going to the emergency room is important and that time for medical interventions should not be delayed.

A heart attack is not that difficult to identify as a crushing and excruciating chest pain that is often described as a vise gripping the heart or as an elephant sitting down on one's chest. However, there are some cases of heart attacks that may be undetected or not even felt by the person having the heart attack. These "silent" heart attacks are considered deadlier since they can display no obvious signs and symptoms, but still continue causing extensive damage to the heart by delaying medical intervention. A great deal of knowledge, skill, and care is required when it comes to dealing with heart attacks, but composure is also a key factor when it comes to handling a heart attack.

Cocktails and More

In this book, we'll be talking about heart attacks or myocardial infarctions, everything about it, including the signs and symptoms of heart attacks, the diagnostic tests used to identify a myocardial infarction, the management for a heart attack, and even the emergency management and the things you should if you see someone having a heart attack or experience a heart attack yourself.

Are you ready to challenge yourself and tackle one of the greatest medical emergencies in the world? Sit back and read on to know more about Heart Attack and its Management.

Chapter 1 - What is a Heart Attack?

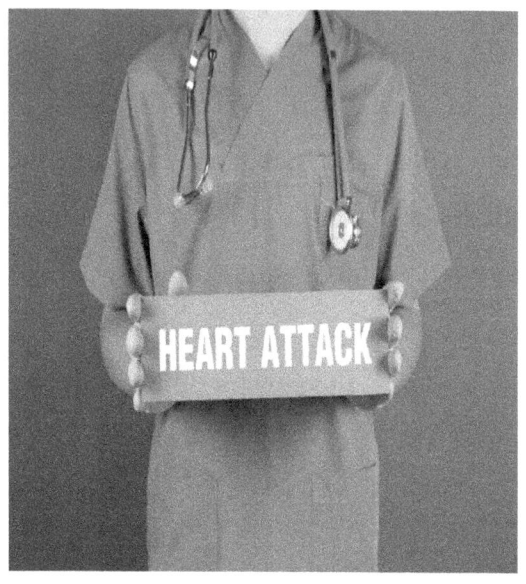

A heart attack, also termed as *myocardial infarction*, basically occurs when the heart doesn't get enough supply of oxygen to serve as its lifeline for its constant workload. The heart is known as an involuntary muscle that never stops working, day in and day out, 24 hours a day, and 7 days a week. When the supply of oxygen is suddenly cut off, the heart muscles can go into arrest and experience tissue damage called "ischemia". The very tiny blood vessels that are latched on to the heart muscle, the coronary arteries, are the ones responsible for supplying the blood for the heart muscles.

A heart attack occurs when there's something wrong with the blood flow in the coronary arteries, slowing down the circulation to the heart muscles and resulting in injury because of the lack of oxygen. Oftentimes, this is due to a blockage in the coronary arteries from the unstable buildup of white blood cells, cholesterol, or fatty plaque deposits.

Chest pain the most common complaint of a person having a heart attack. The chest pain is often described as coming from behind the sternum and may even radiate to the left arm or the left side of the neck. Most people describe this chest pain as vise-like, constricting, or crushing, as if an elephant is sitting down on their chest. Other associated signs and symptoms include shortness of breath, nausea, vomiting, abnormal heart rhythms, sweating, anxiety, and a sense of impending doom. There are also some cases in which heart attacks don't display obvious signs and symptoms. These heart attacks are often termed as "silent" myocardial infarctions and are usually more deadly since it causes the person to delay medical treatment and allow the damage to the heart muscles to worsen as time passes by.

There are several factors that come into play when it comes to the development of a heart attack. These may include a number of cardiovascular conditions, older age, cigarette smoking, increased cholesterol levels, diabetes mellitus, high blood pressure, chronic kidney disease, alcohol intake, and the use of illegal drugs like methamphetamine, cocaine, and heroin.

What makes heart attacks so serious is that they often come without warning, can occur any time of the day, and can occur in almost anyone. This wide range of demographic and incidence of heart attacks among people is what makes heart attacks so life threatening and since it affects the heart, prompt medical treatment is a must to treat the condition. Without taking the person to the emergency room, the person who is having a heart attack may deteriorate because of the increased injury to the heart muscles and it may even result in death.

There are various complications that can result from a heart attack or myocardial infarction. Heart failure can result from the inadequate supply of oxygen that the heart requires, overworking either side of the heart, abnormally increasing in size, and resulting in cardiac damage. Another complication is an abnormal heart rhythm which results from the changes in the conduction of the electrical signals of the heart and bring about even less oxygenation to the body because of the irregular rhythms of the heart. Lastly, another complication that can result from a heart attack is cardiac arrest or the immediate stopping of the heart that can result in death if emergency medical intervention is not done.

Fortunately, there are various treatments available in the management of heart attacks. Throughout the years, modifications and improvements in the healthcare industry and medicine have made it possible to treat heart attacks in the most immediate time and leave with little to no permanent complications after the recovery period for the person who experienced a heart attack. A combination of medications, oxygen therapy, and various care modalities play a key role in the management of heart attacks.

Heart attacks can potentially lead to cardiac arrest – the immediate stopping of the heart. Cardiopulmonary resuscitation or CPR plays a key role in saving the lives of those who suffer from heart attacks, especially those who experience a heart attack in public places. Today, several healthcare institutions offer courses to teach people how to perform CPR correctly and the other things that even those who are not working in the healthcare setting can do to help people who may have experienced a heart attack.

The prognosis for myocardial infarction varies depending on one's overall health, the extent of the cardiac damage due to ischemia, and the different treatment modalities given.

Chapter 2 - Signs and Symptoms of a Heart Attack

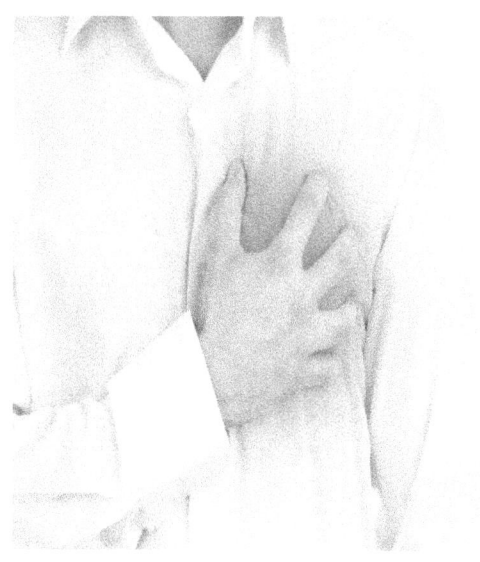

While a heart attack may come as sudden or without warning, the onset of the signs and symptoms are often gradual by nature and rarely instantaneous. It's just that these signs and symptoms are often overlooked as a simple discomfort and the heart attack progresses further without medical intervention. While being a cardiac condition, a myocardial infarction can display a variety of signs and symptoms that mainly affects the heart, the blood circulation, the breathing, and the level of consciousness of the person.

Chest pain the most common complaint of those who experience a heart attack. It is often described as crushing and vise-like, as if an elephant is sitting on your chest and often directed behind the sternum and may radiate to the left arm, the abdomen, the left side of the neck or shoulder. There are also other signs and symptoms when it comes to myocardial infarction and may include the following:

- Crushing chest pain that may radiate to the left arm, neck, or shoulder
- Shortness of breath or dyspnea
- Fatigue
- Diaphoresis or excessive sweating
- A sense of impending doom
- Anxiety
- Light headedness
- Weakness
- Nausea
- Vomiting
- Sleep disturbances
- Palpitations
- Abnormal heart rhythms
- Abnormal pulse rate
- Decreased level of consciousness
- Loss of consciousness

The signs and symptoms of myocardial infarction often come from the intense surge of catecholamines coming from the sympathetic nervous system which is stimulated by the response to pain and the abnormal blood flow coming from the abnormality in the heart muscles due to the ischemic damage that occur in a heart attack.

A decreased or loss of consciousness may also result if there isn't enough blood flowing to the brain and due to cardiogenic shock. Cardiac arrest and death can also occur often due to the development of ventricular fibrillation or other abnormal heart rhythms that can result in the further damage or ischemia to the heart muscles. Other signs and symptoms may arise due to a potential development of pulmonary edema the longer a person experiences a myocardial infarction.

Signs and symptoms may also vary depending on the person as women, the elderly, and those with diabetes may have varying experiences when it comes to heart attacks. Women experience more symptoms when compared to men, usually including dyspnea, weakness, and fatigue. There are also some reports that signs and symptoms like dyspnea, fatigue, and sleep problems may even manifest a month before the ischemic changes occur in the heart muscles.

What's scary about heart attacks is that about a fourth of all myocardial infarctions are silent by nature, exhibiting no chest pain or other signs and symptoms. These silent heart attacks can later be discovered through various diagnostic tests like electrocardiograms and testing the blood enzymes. Silent heart attacks are more common in the elderly and those with diabetes primarily because of the change in the pain threshold.

When these signs and symptoms result in the interruption of the blood flow of the heart which would include conditions like ST Elevation Myocardial Infarction or STEMI, non-ST Elevation Myocardial Infarction or NSTEMI, and unstable angina, the condition is then referred to as Acute Coronary Syndrome or ACS.

Chapter 3 - How to Diagnose a Heart Attack

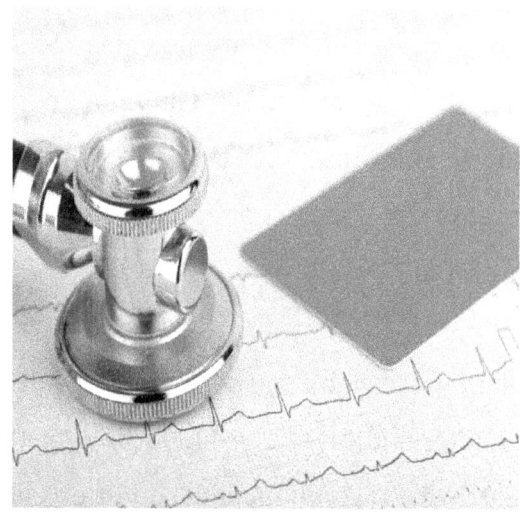

To diagnose a heart attack, a variety of tests is involved in its confirmation. Establishing a diagnosis for myocardial infarction isn't that difficult and it can be done once the patient gets to the emergency room. Typically, a baseline ECG or electrocardiogram is taken to know the rhythm changes in the heart for a person who experienced a heart attack. Blood enzymes are then tested to confirm the occurrence of a heart attack. Other diagnostic tests are also acquired to further establish a strong foundation of diagnosing the heart attack, as well as other correlated health conditions that may contribute to the incidence of the heart attack. Here are just some of the diagnostic tests used to detect and diagnose a heart attack in a patient:

- **Electrocardiogram or 12 Lead ECG**
  ○ Being the mainstay diagnostic test to diagnose a heart attack, an ECG is used to determine the rhythm of the heart, whether it's normal or abnormal, and if there are significant changes in the electrical conduction capacity of the heart

as displayed by the different waves such as the P wave, QRS complex, ST segment, and U wave.

• Creatinine Kinase (CK-MB) test

○ Testing the blood enzyme, CK-MB or creatinine kinase, is vital for the establishing a concrete diagnosis of a heart attack. CK-MB is the earliest indicator of a heart attack and is often tested in cardiac patients, particularly those who are at risk to develop a myocardial infarction. However, CK-MB becomes unreliable when the ischemic damage to the heart is prolonged as it can only detect the early onset of a heart attack.

- **Troponin test**

o   Troponin is another cardiac enzyme that can be tested for those who experienced a heart attack. What makes Troponin stand out is that it is considered as the most accurate cardiac enzyme test to establish a strong diagnosis for a heart attack. It's reliable as it measures the Troponin, a crucial indicator for those with cardiac injury; whether the patient with a heart attack sought consult early or late.

- **Lactate   Dehydrogenase (LDH)**

o   Another cardiac biomarker, lactate dehydrogenase is often used to identify a heart attack during its late phase. LDH is often tested for those patients who have opted to delay medical consultation and the ischemic damage on the heart may already be obvious. At this point, the CK-MB levels may be normal; however, testing the LDH may yield an elevated result.

• **Coronary Angiography**

o   If the various diagnostic tests prove to be inefficient in determining the diagnosis of a heart attack, a coronary angiography may be performed. This is done by inserting a very thin catheter into the blood vessels and a dye is introduced. This is to identify the blood flow into the coronary arteries and see if there is a blockage or obstruction within the coronary arteries which may be the culprit for the heart attack.

- **2D Echocardiogram**

o   An echocardiogram is used to identify the condition of the cardiac walls. For those with heart attack, visible ischemic damage may be detected through an echocardiogram and is often used in various cardiac conditions.

- **Chest X-ray**

o   A chest X-ray may also be performed for patients with myocardial infarction as it may show cardiomegaly or an enlargement of the heart. Prolonged ischemic damage, often due to the delay in seeking medical treatment, for those with a heart attack may cause one or both sides of the heart to fail and enlarge to compensate in the lack of oxygenation, thus resulting in cardiomegaly.

Diagnosing a heart attack involves the use of various tests. With the combination of cardiac enzyme biomarkers, electrocardiogram, and imaging tests, a diagnosis for a heart attack or myocardial infarction can be strongly established.

Physical assessment places utmost importance when it comes to establishing a diagnosis for myocardial infarction. A thorough and accurate assessment, not only for the cardiovascular system, but as well as the other body systems should be done to pinpoint and determine the cause of the chest pain and eliminate other medical conditions that may display similar signs and symptoms.

Routine diagnostic tests are also done to serve as baseline data for those who had a heart attack. A complete blood count, urinalysis, fecalysis, and serum blood tests may be acquired during the course of hospitalization or even upon the arrival of the patient in the emergency room.

One last leg of diagnosing a heart attack is by doing a differential diagnosis which involves the comparison of various signs and symptoms with other conditions that may display similar signs and symptoms. These conditions may include the likes of pulmonary edema, cholecystitis, biliary tract disease, endocarditis, gastric esophageal reflux disease, mitral valve regurgitation, arrhythmias, pancreatitis, and more.

It's important that a strong foundation for a diagnosis of a heart attack is established so that treatment modalities can be specific and target the exact cause of the heart attack. There are times when inadequate assessment can lead to things that are left out, affecting the quality of the management for a patient who had just had a heart attack. Thoroughness and completeness of data during the initial assessment period, including the history and lifestyle habits, is essential to serve as the concrete baseline date for determining a diagnosis for a heart attack.

Chapter 4 - Management of a Heart Attack

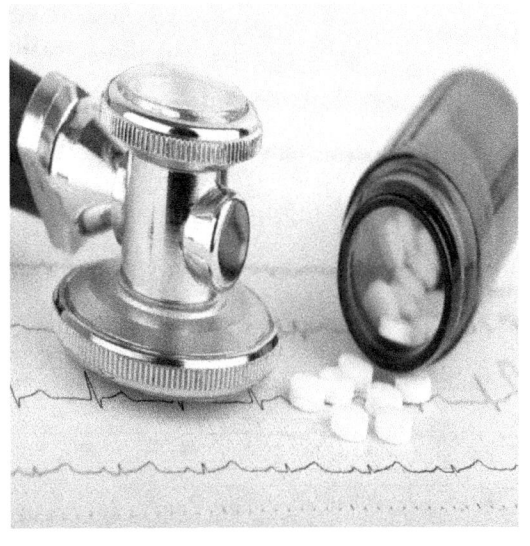

Cardiac conditions often involve the use of medication therapy to aid in the recovery of conditions like atherosclerosis, angina pectoris, and myocardial infarction. While a heart attack may sound threatening and hopeless, managing it is possible and there are various stages when it comes to managing a heart attack.

The goals in managing a heart attack include the relief of pain, restoration of the optimum oxygen supply to the heart, prevention of further damage due to ischemia in the heart, salvage the function of the parts damaged by the ischemia, and prevent any complications that may arise because of the heart attack.

After knowing the different tests and diagnostic procedures to identify the occurrence of a heart attack and establish a concrete diagnosis, it's time to talk about the various treatment modalities and management for a heart attack. Here are some of the treatments involved in managing a heart attack.

- ## Oxygen Therapy

o   In a heart attack, the cardiac muscles experience a lacking supply of oxygen. Because of this, starting oxygen therapy once the patient is taken to the emergency room is important to prevent further ischemic damage to the heart.

- ## Nitroglycerin

o   Just after oxygen, a nitroglycerin patch may be given to the patient who just had a heart attack to lower blood pressure and provide relief of the chest pain. Nitroglycerin improves the coronary blood flow in exchange for lowering the blood pressure, so it is important that precautionary measures be taken before giving nitroglycerin to patients who have had a heart attack.

- ## Anti-Platelets

○ As a precautionary measure, anti-platelets are given to patients with heart attack to prevent the clotting up of blood which may cause further ischemia by blocking the coronary arteries. As a preventive approach, anti-platelets don't necessarily offer a cure, but prevent the incidence of heart attacks in the future. However, anti-platelets are contraindicated if a patient has any bleeding disorders or has any abnormality in their bleeding parameters.

- ## Fibrinolytic Therapy

○ One of the most effective healthcare modalities when it comes to myocardial infarction is the administration of fibrinolytic agents. These agents promote the fibrolysis or the dissolving of a potential clot, may it be a blood clot, fatty deposits, or cholesterol plaques that may have been lodged in the coronary arteries and decrease the blood flow to the cardiac muscles, resulting in ischemic damage to the heart.

• **Anti-hypertensive Agents**

o The presence of high blood pressure or hypertension among patients becomes a huge risk factor in the development of a heart attack. This is the reason why the administration of anti-hypertensive agents like calcium channel blockers, beta blockers, and ACE inhibitors are important to control a patient's blood pressure.

• **Diuretics**

○　　When a potential heart failure starts to develop in a person who had a heart attack, one side or even both sides of the heart may enlarge due to overworking of the heart in an attempt to compensate for the inadequate supply of oxygen to the heart muscles. In this case, diuretics may be administered to reduce the size of the excessively large heart by excreting fluids, as well as decreasing the blood pressure.

• **Cardiac Glycosides**

○　　When there is a clog in the coronary arteries, one side of the heart may tend to overwork itself and further increase the damage. In this case, cardiac glycosides are administered to ensure that doesn't happen. The administration of digoxin (Lanoxin) is one of the mainstay treatment options when it comes to patients who have experienced a heart attack to prevent the enlargement of the heart due to an increased workload. However, extreme care must be observed in the administration of these drugs as it can cause toxicity.

- **Analgesics**

o   One of the main goals in the treatment of a heart attack is to offer relief to chest pain. With the intense characteristic of pain, analgesics may be given to a patient to offer relief. Morphine is considered to be one of the main pain management modalities many years ago and is still used in some healthcare institutions now. However, several studies have shown an increased mortality rate among patients who suffered from heart attack and have taken morphine as an opioid analgesic to manage their pain. Other analgesics that may be administered to patients with myocardial infarction include tramadol and paracetamol.

- **Laxatives**
  - Straining during defecation may increase blood pressure, giving way to another episode of a heart attack. As a preventive measure, laxatives like lactulose may be given to the patient who had suffered from a heart attack.

- **Percutaneous Transluminal Coronary Angiography (PTCA)**
  - When the use of medications has proven to be inefficient or ineffective in dealing with a blockage in the coronary

arteries, a surgical procedure can be done to provide relief of the obstruction. A Percutaneous Transluminal Coronary Angiography or PTCA may be performed. In this procedure, a thin catheter with a balloon on its tip is inserted into the affected coronary artery. Visualization may be achieved through the injection of a dye and the blockage which can be due to fatty deposits or a blood clot is then compressed as the balloon on the tip of the catheter is inflated.

• Coronary Artery Bypass Graft (CABG)

o When all other treatment modalities have failed in removing the blockage in the coronary artery, a Coronary Artery Bypass Graft or CABG may be done. In this surgical procedure,

41

removing the blood clot or fatty plaque on the coronary arteries is withheld and another path is made by the use of a graft, often from another blood vessel, to provide another way for the blood to flow. This ensures adequate perfusion of blood to the heart even when there is still the presence of a blockage that may not be removed due to the high risks of its removal or the difficulty in removing the blockage itself.

• Cardiopulmonary Resuscitation (CPR)

o   When a heart attack results in cardiac arrest or the immediate stopping of the heart's pumping ability, cardiopulmonary resuscitation or CPR must be done immediately. The chest compressions in CPR simulate the powerful pumping of the heart to ensure optimal perfusion rate throughout the body and to make sure that the vital organs get adequate blood flow. The brain can only survive for a few minutes without oxygen and it can only be acquired through the blood. It's important that CPR is done in the timeliest manner upon the detection of a cardiac arrest and even those who are not working in the medical field can perform it. Today, there are several institutions that provide training in CPR for various ages, from adolescents up to adults.

- **Cardiac Defibrillation**

o When a heart attack results in a fatal arrhythmia, defibrillation may be done to regulate the heart rhythm and return it to normal. Cardiac defibrillation administers a set amount of electricity to the heart through the use of special pads in order to return the heart rhythm to normal. Special precautionary measures are observed when administering defibrillation or shock to a patient who had a heart attack and training is done for those who will administer shock.

The various treatment modalities for heart attacks strongly depend upon the diagnosis of myocardial infarction, specifically its type. STEMI and NSTEMI have different management options and it should be specified which type a heart attack is during the initial assessment of a patient in the emergency room. Achieving the goals in a patient with a heart attack namely, the relief of chest pain, the prevention of further damage due to ischemia, and to salvage the damaged cardiac muscles, can be attained with these interventions.

Chapter 5 - Preventing a Heart Attack

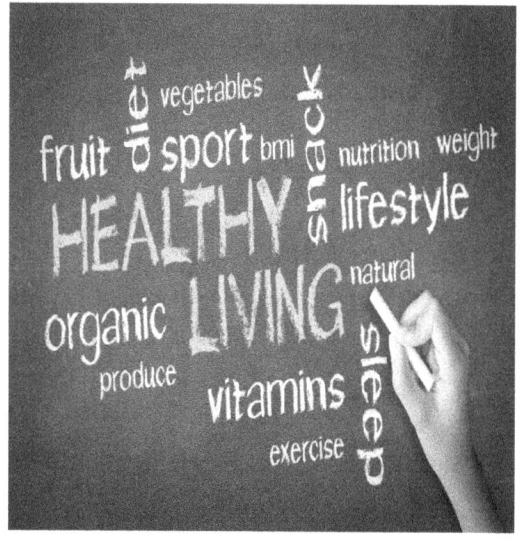

While there are various treatment options for a heart attack, the most effective way in stopping a heart attack is to stop it from happening in the first place. Prevention is better than cure, as they say. Sure, there may be medications and procedures to help in relieving the chest pain and preventing further ischemic damage during a heart attack; however, that doesn't change the fact that the prevention of a heart attack is way better. Taking a look at the different risk factors that increase the likelihood of a heart attack is crucial to prevent its occurrence in the first place.

Cessation of smoking is one of the primary lifestyle changes one has to make in order to prevent the occurrence and recurrence of a heart attack. That's because the different chemicals in cigarette and tobacco cause the vasoconstriction of the blood vessels which increases the blood pressure, further increasing the risk for a heart attack. Quitting smoking is important in preventing the case of a heart attack and health teachings on its benefits should be further stressed out and explained to a patient who had a previous heart attack or any correlating cardiac condition.

Eating a proper diet is also essential as buildup of excess fat and cholesterol further increases the risk of fatty deposits to become lodged in the arteries, particularly in the coronary arteries. A healthy and balanced diet is important when it comes to preventing the incidence of a heart attack. One's diet should include a rich amount of fruits and vegetables with a limited amount of fats. This reduces the risk of fatty deposits in the coronary arteries, preventing a potential heart attack or even other cardiovascular conditions.

Cocktails and More

Regular exercise is another key factor in the lifestyle changes that one can make to prevent the occurrence of a heart attack. Exercise helps promote a healthy heart and reduces the risk for the development of cardiac conditions like angina pectoris, atherosclerosis, and myocardial infarction. With the consistent exertion of effort through regular exercise, the heart gets adequate work and becomes more resistant to fatigue and it also promotes a healthy perfusion or circulation of blood throughout the body.

Reducing alcohol intake may also prevent the occurrence of a heart attack. Studies have shown that excessive consumption of alcohol increase the likelihood of a person to develop cardiovascular problems like high blood pressure, contributing to the development of a heart attack. Liver problems may also arise with excessive alcohol intake which can also contribute to the deterioration of the blood vessels' condition, further increasing the risk of a heart attack.

Conclusion

A heart attack is considered to be one of the top emergency cases in the healthcare setting. It comes without warning and oftentimes, the signs and symptoms are incredibly alarming, especially to the patient. As ischemic damage occurs to the heart, the cardiac muscles may gain irreversible damage if prompt medical intervention is not given. However, all is not lost as there are various ways to manage a heart attack and save the life of a person who had suffered from a heart attack.

There are various risk factors that play their role in increasing the likelihood for the development of a heart attack. Among them, lifestyle habits seem to have more impact as cigarette smoking, excessive alcohol intake, insufficient exercise, an unhealthy diet, and a sedentary lifestyle provide a bigger impact in the development of heart attacks and other cardiac conditions. However, other health problems may predispose a person to having a heart attack which can include the likes of atherosclerosis, high blood pressure, angina pectoris, increased serum cholesterol levels, and more.

The complications associated with heart attacks are alarming because they can be fatal or leave irreversible damage over the few months after the recovery period from a heart attack. Complications like heart failure, pulmonary embolism, mitral valve regurgitation, abnormal heart rhythms, angina pectoris, and a recurrence of the heart attack.

Management of a heart attack involves providing relief of the chest pain, preventing further damage to the heart due to ischemia, and saving the parts of the heart that sustained ischemic damage due to the heart attack. Most often, the management of a heart attack involves the use of medications to relieve signs and symptoms, as well as promoting adequate perfusion to the body and helping the heart compensate for the decreased level of oxygen circulating in the body.

Surgical interventions like PTCA and CABG are done as the last leg of managing a heart attack to remove the obstruction in the coronary arteries and ensure that there is adequate perfusion to the heart muscles. When a heart attack leads to a fatal arrhythmia, defibrillation may be done to regulate the heart rhythm and return it to normal.

Through the numerous treatment options available for those who have experienced a heart attack, prevention is still the strongest intervention one can make. Because of how serious a heart attack can become, preventing it from happening in the first place is the most effective way to manage it. Engaging in healthy lifestyle habits like cessation of cigarette or tobacco smoking, limiting alcohol intake, eating a healthy diet, and getting regular exercise is a must if you want to prevent heart attacks from occurring.

Hopefully, this eBook has provided you with everything that you needed to know about heart attacks and how to manage a heart attack, even if you're away from the hospital. Recognizing the signs and symptoms of a heart attack or even an impending heart attack is important if you want to save the life of a family member, a loved one, or even yourself.

But in its entirety, it is important to keep calm and compose yourself once you see someone having a heart attack or if you experience one yourself. This gives you a clear mind on what are the things that you need to do and devise ways on how to control the chest pain and prevent further damage of the heart due to the ischemic changes in the coronary arteries.

Be calm, be alert, and be ready – that's what it takes to handle this cardiac emergency that is the vise of the heart.